LIVING THE CHIEF LIFE

How to Nourish Yourself for Optimal
Health, Well-Being, and Quality of Life

Stacey Lee Turner

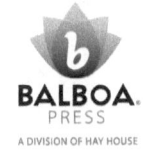

BALBOA.
PRESS

A DIVISION OF HAY HOUSE

Balboa Press books may be ordered through booksellers or by contacting:

Balboa Press
A Division of Hay House
1663 Liberty Drive
Bloomington, IN 47403
www.balboapress.com.au
1 (877) 407-4847

Print information available on the last page.

ISBN: 978-1-5043-1605-7 (sc)
ISBN: 978-1-5043-1606-4 (e)

Balboa Press rev. date: 01/21/2019

CONTENTS

INTRODUCTION

Hello and welcome to *Living The Chief Life*. A "how to" guide to assist you in nourishing yourself for optimal health, well-being and quality of life using a holistic and inclusive approach involving physical, mental, emotional and spiritual aspects.

I have been a practising dietitian since I graduated from Sydney University in 2009 with first-class honours, majoring in nutrition and dietetics. My passion for food and how it helps people be the best and most healthy version of themselves has led me on a wonderful journey of learning and discovery (both for myself and others). This has inspired and guided me in developing the Real Food Experience, which led to the inception of The Chief Life. The Real Food Experience was a 30-day lifestyle program I created in 2012, when I ran my own gym in Maroubra, Sydney, Australia, that allowed me to guide and assist my members, and members of other gyms around Australia, to improve their health, well-being and quality of life through food and lifestyle changes. The Chief Life is a full-service holistic wellness operation, started in April 2015, founded by my now husband and me as a way for us to reach more people across the globe with our knowledge and tools in nutrition, health, and well-being. We take a holistic approach to health and lifestyle and have a strong desire to share this with as many people as possible through our educational tools, personalised meal plan templates, blogs, podcasts, recipe video on social media, and in person at our wellness retreats. The Real Food Experience grew into the Chief Up Nutrition and Lifestyle Program and other health programs we run through The Chief Life online and face-to-face platforms.

This book is a collection of highlights (or as I like to call them, gold nuggets) and useful information / knowledge bombs that I (along with my amazing husband, Matty Turner) have gathered together and developed over our years in the health industry. We are excited to share these with you in the hope that it will help you, and/or your loved ones, on your health and fitness journey too!

I have worked with thousands of awesome humans through my career as a dietitian and found so much success with each and every motivated person who took on our principles and allowed him or herself permission to succeed. Even those who only followed some of our recommendations still achieved positive change and benefits for their overall health and well-being through learning new tools and approaches to food, diet, health, and a positive lifestyle.

Living The Chief Life can be used as either a four-week detox (defined as a cleansing of the body to help remove toxins and unwanted chemicals from your system to increase health and well-being) or more gradually, as a four-month longer-term lifestyle change. All the essential and baseline tools are provided here for you as the gold standard for methods I have found to work best for the majority of people. If you follow this guide, you will likely achieve the results you're after. However, you get to decide for yourself how hardcore you go. Following 50 per cent of the principles will still allow you to see positive changes in the right direction. But the results will match the effort—so 50 per cent effort will give you 50 per cent results.

Another way to think about it is whether you want to be a gold medallist, a silver medallist, a bronze medallist, or maybe not even on the podium. Although, I hope that if you are taking steps to improve your health, you at least want to be standing on the podium. If you follow these principles as close to 100 per cent as possible, you take the gold. Follow 80 to 90 per cent of them, and you'll be winning the silver. And 60 to 70 per cent will earn you a bronze medal. If it seems more realistic to make smaller incremental changes, little by little—so this works for you long term and you find your balance—then start with that. As you start to see the benefits of what this way of life can do for you and how it will make you *feel*, it'll get easier to start to make even more positive changes.

The Chief Life will help you to:

C – Find *clarity* around food *choices*, giving you *confidence*.
H – Know the h*ow* to, whether it's the when, what, and how much or the why behind the science, giving you o*ptions* to help to show you the w*ay*!
I – *Inspire* others, as well as *inspiring* yourself to continue to make changes to be the best version of yourself you can be.
E – *Evolve* to *elevate* your life and *engage* you with your body and mind so you can continue to grow and learn.
F – Gain *freedom*. Whether you want to save money, time, or energy, The Chief Life will give you the tools to gain back *freedom* in all of these areas and more!

MODULE 1

Clean It Up!

Activity 1.1: Where Are You On Your Health Journey Right Now? Self-Assessment and Analysis

Before we start your journey, it's important to assess your current status by checking in with your current food intake, exercise program, and daily routine. Complete the following questionnaire so you can choose the best plan of action to reach your goals right now.

Name: Date:

Gender: Age: DOB:

Job title: Work hours per day (average):

Livingarrangement:

Health issues:

Height: Weight: BMI (body mass index):   Body fat percentage:

Waist girth (measure in line with your belly button, using a measuring tape):

Hip girth (measure in line with the widest part of your butt, using a measuring tape):
Waist-to-hip ratio (waist girth divided by hip girth):
Goal: fat loss / improve energy / gain muscle (Circle one only.)

> Need help with deciding which step of the journey you're currently on? Think of it as a step-by-step process. If you currently have any excess fat mass you'd like to shift, start with fat loss. If your body composition (defined here as muscle-to-fat ratio) is healthy and where you want it to be, your focus should be to improve energy. And if you're a string bean, struggling to put on weight/muscle or you train at a high volume due to being an athlete, you're probably looking to gain muscle as your main focus right now. Note: eating this way should improve energy regardless after a few weeks but if you have another focus right now, make that the main focus as your energy will improve as a by-product.

Goal weight circumference, and/or body fat percentage?

> If you're not sure, use the guidance in the analysis section to help you with setting realistic and health-related goals. We encourage you to focus less on aesthetics

(what you looks like) and more on your health (how you feel and your health markers).

Do you currently prepare/cook any meals at home and take them to work/out with you? Yes / No

Do you have any known food allergies/ intolerances? Yes / No

If yes, explain:

Do you eat regular meals throughout the day? Yes / No

Have you made any changes to more healthful choices in the last month? Yes / No

Are you ready to make change to commit to your health? Yes / No

How to analyse your answers

If your job is sedentary, are you taking regular standing breaks to walk around the office and get some fresh air?

If you work more than eight hours a day, are you taking regular breaks to eat balanced nutritious meals and drink plenty of water?

Do you have access to a fully functioning kitchen within your living arrangements? And are you in complete control of what you eat? In other words, do you cook the food or is someone cooking for you? If someone is cooking for you, is he or she open to cooking something different?

Health issues may require you to work more closely with an allied health professional, such as a dietitian, nutritionist, naturopath, or functional medicine doctor.

BMI (body mass index)

Don't use BMI as the be-all and end-all. It's best to use this along with other health measures and markers because it doesn't take into consideration your body composition (again that is, your muscle-to-fat ratio). To calculate your BMI, take your total body weight in kilograms (for example, 65 kg), divided by your height in metres squared (for example, 1.63 × 1.63). So for this example, BMI = 65 / (1.63 × 1.63) = 65 / 2.66 = 24.4.

The healthy range for BMI is considered to be between 20 and 25, with anything less than 20 considered underweight and anything greater than 25 being into the overweight/obese realm. Now, my opinion is that BMI cannot be taken as a stand-alone measure of health because, during the course of my time working in the health and fitness industry, I have seen healthy people with a BMI greater than 25 due to the high level of muscle they have. This means that BMI should not be the only measure used. BMI used in conjunction with waist and hip circumference measurements are essential in determining whether you're in the healthy range or not. Please see the next few sections for more information on how to assess these circumferences and use them to calculate your waist-to-hip ratio.

Body fat percentage

This is the percentage of fat mass you have compared to your total body weight. Body fat percentage is a very useful measure of how your body composition changes beneath the skin when you make alterations to your diet, lifestyle, and environment. Seeing your body fat percentage decrease and your muscle mass increase is a great way to know that your new health program is moving you in the right direction. The gold standards for determination of body fat percentage are a DEXA (dual energy X-ray absorptiometry) scan or a BIA (bio-impedance analysis) scan, both of which provide fairly accurate readings. However, like all measurements concerning the human body, they can still be affected by water / hydration level, time of day, salt concentration, sleep, stress, and whether you've eaten a higher fat meal. So it's important to understand but not be fixated on the numbers. How you feel is super important. And if you are making better choices the majority of the time, you are likely on the right track.

Eating and living for optimal health is a long-term change, not a short-term fix. So don't expect to do a crash diet for four weeks and see massive changes in your body composition at the end. We need to take all factors on board and make positive change in all areas, not just with food but also with mindset, sleep, breathing, movement, outside time and hydration. Health is a consistency game, and we need both physical and mental health to really thrive.

We're in this for the long haul.

The ranges for female body fat percentage are:

Essential fat	10%–13%
Very lean	14%–20%
Lean	21%–25%
Normal	26%–31%
Overweight	32%–39%
Obese	40% and over

The ranges for male body fat percentage are:

Essential fat	2%–5%
Very lean	6%–13%
Lean	14%–17%
Normal	18%–22%
Overweight	23%–29%
Obese	30% and over

As you can see, there is a vast difference between male and female ranges. This has a lot to do with optimising health. If body fat is too low for a female, it affects our ability to function at our best due to changes in hormone balance, brain function, mood, menstrual cycle, and so on.

Waist circumference

For a male, a healthy waist is 94 cm or less. For a female, it's 80 cm or less. Having a waist circumference higher than these numbers with respect to your gender may increase your risk of metabolic diseases.

Waist-to-hip ratio: Waist circumference / hip circumference

A ratio of less than 0.9 for guys and less than 0.8 for women is ideal. This is calculated by dividing your waist circumference with your hip circumference.

Your goal

If your goal is fat loss, follow the guidelines for creating a fat loss (FL) meal plan. For improved energy and performance use improved energy (IE) meal plan guidelines. And for putting on some size, use gain muscle (GM) meal plan guidelines in the meal planning section when you are calculating your daily intake.

If you don't currently cook or prepare your own food, you may need to carve time in your day or week for this to happen. Perhaps sit down with your family to figure out a schedule where everyone takes meal preparation in turns or everybody helps out. If your life is too busy at the moment, it's time to look at your priorities and add food preparation close to the top of the list. In order to function at your best, you have to put your health first. If you let this drop to the bottom of the list (or off the list completely), your health will suffer and you may get sick, with quality of life being decreased. It's unlikely you will be thriving or working at your optimal performance. If not now, when? Don't put your health on the backburner, you get to choose how and if you take positive steps forward today! I believe in you, now believe in yourself and you'll be surprised at what you can achieve. Give yourself permission to succeed.

Check in with how you're spending your time. An hour spent on social media might be better spent on food planning and preparation. If it's more down to working around the family schedule, commit to doing meal prep early on a Sunday morning whilst the rest of the family is sleeping so you can get some uninterrupted prep time. It's actually really nice "you" time—put on some music or listen to a podcast, then chop up and cook the veggies so they're ready for the week ahead, whilst you throw some meat in the slow cooker!

If you have known allergies or intolerances, *do not eat these foods! Ever!* If you know a food causes you discomfort, whether it's gut discomfort, sinus issues, rashes, gas, snoring, lethargy (tiredness), brain fog, or just a general feeling of "bleurgh," that food does not allow you to be the most healthful version of yourself and may have detrimental effects on your long-term health. For example, eating ice cream when you know you are lactose intolerant will damage the lining of your gut, stopping you from being able to absorb nutrients from your food properly. Over many years, this abuse may lead to bowel cancer or other gut issues. Listen to your body and be aware of signs and symptoms to discover which foods allow you to function at your absolute best and which should be avoided because they lead you further from your goals and further from feeling like an 11 out of 10 on your energy scale (1 being low energy, 10 being super high)!

Ideally, you should be eating at least two to three times a day, and perhaps even up to five or six times. This will be dependent on your schedule and what suits you as an individual, but we do encourage most people to start with three meals and two snacks spread evenly throughout the day so that you can find your new equilibrium, and adjusting after the first four to six weeks if needed.

If you have already started to make some changes, that is amazing. It means you are in a great headspace to start

Living The Chief Life and tackling your health and well-being. You have taken *action*!

If you are ready to commit to making changes to your health, fantastic. If not, remember that mindset is part of your health, so we can start working on this area of your health too. Shifting mindset and getting you on your own side might be the first step to starting this journey for you. Without you backing yourself, it's going to be a much harder process to want to make these changes or even be able to stay focused on *why* you are doing it in the first place. There's more about this in chapter nine, "The Right Focus," which addresses mindset. For now, consider taking some time to reflect by writing in a journal; attempt to ascertain some of the things that might be blocking you from allowing yourself to prioritise your health. You have to want this.

2

The Basics: When, What, and How Much

I like to keep things simple. It's much better to focus on core principles and philosophies, rather than on a set of strict rules that you must follow, such as a meal plan exactly as it's written to the letter. This is unrealistic and unsustainable. What we encourage is using the following basic ideas to help guide you as to how to live The Chief Life in order to feel and function at your best.

Being 100 per cent on track does not mean following a meal plan. It means living by a code. The rule of three is that code: Eat all three macronutrients (defined as a nutrient needed by the body in larger amounts) every three to five hours, in close to a third of each macronutrient. This chapter explains this rule a bit further.

When, what, and how much are key pieces to think about when you are eating for optimal health, well-being and improved quality of life.

When

Eating every three to five hours is the goal. But your daily routine will determine when you can slot your meals and snacks in. Make it work with your current schedule so it is easier to stick to. This is a good starting point to allow your body to get used to eating regularly, keeping your hormones balanced and your body fuelled correctly. Once you have followed this for between four to six weeks, you can start to tweak it based on preferences and circadian rhythms. (Check out *The Chief Life podcast* episodes 40 and 75 with Dr. Michael Breus, the sleep doctor of America for more info on sleep cycles, chronotypes, and the best time of day to start eating based on your chronotype).

For example, if you wake up at 5:00 a.m., your eating schedule might look something like this:

Breakfast – 5:30 a.m.
Snack – 8:30 a.m.
Lunch – 12:30 p.m.
Snack – 3:30 p.m.
Dinner – 7:30 p.m.

Aim to have a snack or breakfast to start your day when you feel ready to eat and then every three to five hours throughout the day.

If you train first thing in the morning, you can either train on an empty stomach (preferable if your goal is fat loss) or try having a small snack before training and breakfast after training (better for improving energy balance and gaining muscle). Some people prefer to fast and eat later, around mid-morning or even lunchtime. This is fine and is personal preference (as well as chronotype dependent), but you'll still need to prioritise getting your daily energy intake of food in, even if you're consuming it during a smaller window.

Write your schedule below with meal or snack name and time:

What

The type or quality of food we eat is important, not only for getting the best nutrients for our body but to give us the best fuel and combination of macronutrients (macros). The macronutrients we need every time we eat are protein, carbohydrate, and fat, which should be eaten as a complete puzzle at every meal *and* snack. In other words, we need a portion of protein, a portion of carbohydrate, and a portion of fat *every* time we eat. If we don't, our energy levels won't remain constant due to our hormones being out of balance.

Protein foods

Proteins include any animal foods—meat, fish and shellfish, poultry and eggs, and dairy (be aware that dairy may also be a carbohydrate/protein combination food, more on dairy later)—and the vegetarian / plant-based protein options like soy, tofu, tempeh, hemp, nutritional yeast, buckwheat, black rice, spirulina, legumes, and beans. Aim for organic and whole foods as much as possible for best quality and health outcomes.

Carbohydrate foods

Carbohydrates are anything that grows in the ground or on a tree. This includes all fruit and water-based non-starchy vegetables and tubers / root vegetables, as well as less processed naturally gluten free grain options like rice, quinoa, buckwheat. (It also includes all the man-made processed stuff that we're going to choose to steer away from for a plethora of reasons, including their high sugar content, ability to cause chronic inflammation in the body, and highly addictive nature with no nutritive benefits. Think bread, pasta, cereals, condiments, and confectionary and baked goods—essentially, anything with added sugar, E-numbers, and ingredients your great-grandparents wouldn't recognise.)

Fat foods

This group is a mix of fruit and nutlike food items, including but not limited to avocados; olives; coconut (any form apart from coconut water, as this counts as a carbohydrate); oils, preferably olive or coconut for cooking, as seed oils are high in pro-inflammatory omega-6; nuts and seeds; and other oils – like avocado or macadamia – to use as dressings after cooking/plating.

How much

This will be different for everyone. It is based on your gender, size, health conditions / current health status, job, and exercise level, as well as your current goal (fat loss, energy balance, or muscle gain). A great place to start is a chief-approved plate as shown in the image that follows.

A chief-approved plate with all three macronutrients (chicken mango avocado salsa). Start making your own by including a palm-size protein, filling your plate with vegetables, and adding a spoon or two of starchy foods with a sprinkle of good fats:

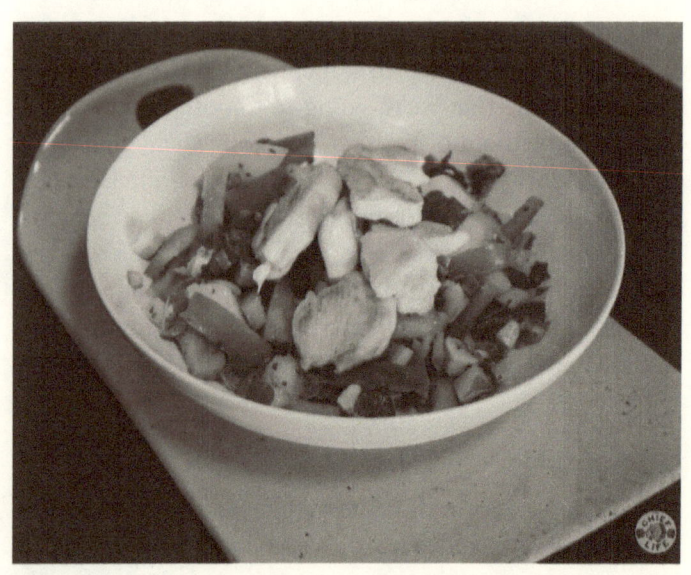

Activity 2.1: Draw Your Current Plate

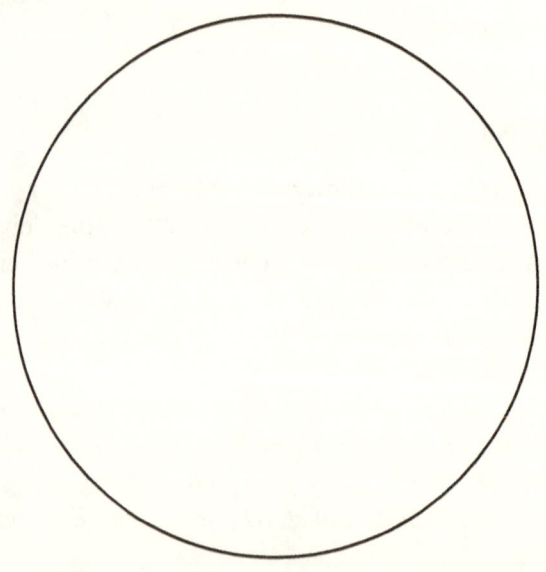

Now make some notes about the changes that need to be made to your current plate to get it looking a bit more like the chief-approved plate from the photo with the chicken mango avocado salsa. Do you need less or more protein, less processed carbs and more plant based carbs, more good fats or less of the unfavourable fats?

Beliefs

Where does your current belief system around food come from? Often we learn these behaviours as kids (from school or our families) or from research we might have done later in life. However, have you ever stopped to question where your thoughts and feelings around what is good for us and what is not so good actually come from? Maybe it's time to analyse these beliefs and even start to challenge some of them. A good friend of mine, Ryan Drake, brought this to my attention as he was proofreading the first draft of this book, and it made a lot of sense to me. Now, when I think about the way I eat at this point in my life, I know my decisions are moulded from the education, research, and study I have done since graduating with my nutrition degree and working within the industry for many years. If I think back to how I ate as a child, teenager and even university student, my habits have changed drastically for the better, and I am a healthier, happier human being because of it.

Take some time to reflect on and maybe even journal how you ate when you were growing up, how your eating pattern has changed over the years, and your thoughts about your plate back then versus now. It might help you to see why you have formed certain habits and how you can shift your belief system if it needs shifting at all. For example, a dear friend of mine, Dean Fogarty, used to be a software engineer, which led to a desk job requiring long periods of concentration at a keyboard. This resulted in irregular eating—just what was available close by. There were a handful of times when he *forgot* to eat because he was engrossed in a problem. So it is worth considering how eating patterns change as you move from school to university/study to work. Maybe once you acknowledge the habits you've created, you'll be able to make changes if needed. Maybe your family has certain traditions that are ingrained in you but might not be as favourable in terms of your health. Starting to find more favourable ways to create these recipes or maybe decreasing the frequency you choose to have them is a good start. If you are similar to Dean in forgetting to it, it might be worth setting an alarm to remind you to step away from your desk at certain times of the day to have a meal or snack in a different environment where you can enjoy and fully digest the nutrients from your food.

How to Get Started

Activity 3.1: Goal setting

Now you have the basics, it's time to get personal and set some goals. Goal setting is an integral part of planning any change to your lifestyle and, if done well, can really make or break your chance of success!

Goals should be SMART! This acronym is really useful for ensuring your goals are specific, measurable, achievable, relevant, and time-bound. For example, I will decrease my waist circumference by 2 cm in four weeks. Another more performance-related goal could be, I will decrease my 5-km run time by three minutes in four weeks. Your goal doesn't have to be body measurement-related or gym/exercise-related. It could be to decrease your "7 Pillars of Health" score by 4 points over four weeks (see module 3, chapter eight "Dial It Up and Dial It In" for more about the 7 Pillars). Write down your health related and performance related goals below now.

Whatever you choose your overall health or performance goals to be, make sure you *write them down* with pen and paper. Don't just write your goals here in your *Living The Chief Life* book; write your goals on a goals sheet you place on your fridge or bedroom wall, where you will see it daily as a reminder of what you want to achieve and by when. Use your questionnaire to help set these goals; if your waist is greater than 80 cm for a female or 94 cm for a male, you might set a goal to decrease it (to decrease risk of developing metabolic diseases).

My health goal is:

My performance goal is:

This is also a great time to consider making some lifestyle changes. You will be making a big effort with your nutrition, training and health over the next four weeks to three months, so it makes sense to inspect all areas that will have an influence on your overall health and fitness results. Consider coffee and alcohol intake, sleep length and quality, current stressors in your life, and chill time for yourself. If you've been trying to quit smoking, now's the time! Choose decreasing or removing coffee and alcohol *or* ensuring you get into bed at a certain time each night to allow for a minimum of six hours sleep but ideally seven and a half hours. Avoid screens prior to sleep *or* decrease stress at work by spending less time there or by increasing your downtime and doing more things that you enjoy. *Or* finally kick that smoking habit once and for all! These are just a few examples. Maybe start with one at a time so it's less overwhelming. The 7 Pillars of Health (chapter eight) will help you with these lifestyle changes later on in the process as well.

My first lifestyle change for right now is:

Write up your health and performance goals and lifestyle change on your goals sheet and attach a calendar so you can tick off every day you manage to allow yourself to stay on your path to success. Give yourself permission to succeed— *allow yourself to succeed*! You are doing something for *you*, so be selfish. You deserve this, and you should allow yourself the love and respect you are worthy of to put yourself first when it comes to your health.

Being selfish is not negative. Think of it as self-care (if selfish brings negative connotations for you) or redefine the word. If you fill up your own cup first and be the best version of yourself you can be, you'll have a lot more to give to those around you who you love and care about. By revamping your nutrition, fitness, health, and overall well-being, you'll ensure that life is much more enjoyable. We are so blessed to get this chance in this body, so we might as well make the most of it. Have the respect for yourself to look after your body; it is a temple. You only have one so you should allow yourself to look after it as best you can.

Remember, food is fuel—not a privilege. And by choosing foods that fuel, nurture and nourish you, you'll be the happiest and most full-of-life version of yourself possible! Definitely still find joy in eating, but work to find joy in eating the things that make you feel good health wise and decrease your risk of disease and discomfort later in life. Prevention is *the best* medicine.

Now that your goals are set, you need to decide how often you will check in with yourself. I like to use weekly or monthly check-ins, as it gets me into a routine. But figure out what works best for you and stick to your routine.

My next self-check-in date is:

Record this in your diary or calendar as an appointment with a reminder and make it a priority!

Meal planning

It's great knowing the what and the why of eating for health and improved quality of life, but now we need the nitty-gritty details (the how to) to put together a plan that fits your life and gets you to your goals.

Once you have your meal timing aligned with your routine and have decided upon a couple of staple breakfast, lunch, dinner, and snack options (feel free to check out the recipe and meal plan ideas in the appendix section), it is time to write yourself a meal plan.

This doesn't mean you have to follow your plan like it's set in stone. Instead, we are putting into practice the 3 P's of successful nutrition—planning, purchasing, and prepping/preparation.

With a system in place, it will be easier to remember all the foods you're meant to eat, at what time, and in what amounts. Beginning with a plan is essential. Over time, as your meal choices become familiar habits, you won't need to write down the weekly plan because it will become your new routine. You'll be able to speedily and easily create meals and snacks on the fly as you go, using our principles.

Success in planning is planning to succeed, so get to it! Use the empty meal plan included in this book to put together a rough guide for your next week ahead. There are suggested meal plans in the appendix section, so feel free to take a peak. Remember to swap out foods you might not like and change portion sizes for your goals and current health status.

Once you have written your meal plan, you can now take the next step—*purchasing*. It's time to go food shopping. Create a full shopping list with all the non-perishable food items you need for the week that you can stock up on (like non fruit and vegetable items). Then maybe add perishables for only the first two to three days. Keep in mind that you'll be doing regular food prep at least twice a week to help set you up for success and ease for staying on track with the plan. An hour or two in the kitchen on a Sunday and maybe twenty to thirty minutes on a Wednesday or Thursday as a top-up day will help you to stay on top of your game. Day by day is achievable but requires a lot more prep time than is really necessary. It just depends on your schedule and work-life balance. Once you have your shopping list, either order online or head to the local markets / fruit and veg store and butchers/ fishmongers to buy all of your delicious and nutritious food items for the first few days of your plan.

Now it's time for the third P. Go home and *prep*. Chop, cook, and box up all the veggies and meat you can, even if it's only prepping for breakfast, snacks, and lunch tomorrow whilst you're cooking dinner for that night. This way, you will be one step ahead and will have easy-to-grab-and-eat meals and snacks for the day ahead. This decreases the risk of straying from our principles and also helps you keep your energy levels balanced. In addition it will keep you satisfied. It will also hopefully prevent you from eating the less favourable food items that aren't part of a healthful outcome. These less favourable foods nearly always find a way to sneak in if we're not fully prepared and our hunger gets the better of us. But if you already have your meals and snacks with you, you'll be less likely to make less favourable choices.

Activity 3.2: Build Your Own Meal Plan (examples are given in the appendix at the back of this book)

Breakfast: Idea 1

Protein	Carbohydrates	Fats

Breakfast: Idea 2

Protein	Carbohydrates	Fats

Morning snack: Idea 1

Protein	Carbohydrates	Fats

Morning snack: Idea 2

Protein	Carbohydrates	Fats

Lunch: Idea 1

Protein	Carbohydrates	Fats

Lunch: Idea 2

Protein	Carbohydrates	Fats

Afternoon snack: Idea 1

Protein	Carbohydrates	Fats

Afternoon snack: Idea 2

Protein	Carbohydrates	Fats

Dinner: Idea 1

Protein	Carbohydrates	Fats

Dinner: Idea 2

Protein	Carbohydrates	Fats

Use these options to alternate or eat one option for two to three days in a row and then switch to the other option for two to three days to make prep easier.

Tracking progress

It is important to keep a record of your numbers and measurements so you can watch your successes week to week and month to month. Doing so will keep you accountable and allow you to assess whether you need to tweak your plan along the way. Remember, if you only follow your plan 50 per cent of the time, you will only see 50 per cent results. So ask yourself, "How much do I want this?" And remind yourself why you want to make a change. That will hopefully help you to stay on track. Print this page out and stick it up on your fridge, bedroom wall, or in your bathroom where you will remember to use it on the allocated day. We recommend weekly to be most effective!

What is your long-term goal? (Three to six months; remember, this is a lifestyle change, not a quick fix.)

(For example, "Health: Decrease waist to below 80 cm if female, 94 cm if male within three months" *or* "Performance: Increase back squat by 10 kg in three months")

What is your SMART goal?

(Specific, measurable, achievable, relative, and time-bound; specific goals are much more likely to produce specific results, just as vague goals will give you vague results)

(For example, "Exercise weekdays at 6:00 a.m." *versus* "Exercise this week")

How will you feel if you achieve this goal?

How will you feel if you *don't* achieve this goal? (This is finding your "pain point," you will be more likely to succeed if you know what you're trying to avoid!)

What is the date you would like to achieve this goal by?

What advice would you give to yourself if you were a high-performance coach?

How do you plan to get there? (It won't happen without an action plan, so write some steps below to help you achieve it.)

(For example, "1. Shop twice a week. 2. Make an appointment with myself for food prep on Sundays and Wednesdays. 3. Check in with The Chief Life Members Page on Facebook—or a friend—daily to report your success in sticking to the plan 90 per cent or more." *Or* "1. Squat twice a week, increasing the weight by 1.25 kg each side each week as long as technique is good. 2. Do a proper warm up before training. 3. Do two minutes of stretching my hips and glutes per day).

Action plan:

How will you stay accountable?

Keep track by choosing one day a week or month to take your measurements and/or observe performance improvements and record them in the following table. It's also a good idea to take note of a positive change you have achieved this week or month. Set a reminder in your phone for your next check-in date with yourself. See first row of table for an example of how to complete.

Progress Chart (Are you on or off track?)

Date	Weight	Waist	Hips	BMI	Body Fat %	Performance	Positive Note	7 Pillars Score (Chapter 8)
Example Dec. 4, 2017	61.9 kg	69 cm	97 cm	24.4	15.7%	back squat: 90 kg x 3	slept eight hours/night	12

Not All Foods Are Created Equal. Food quality is extremely important.

When thinking of food, most people will take it at face value. You go to the supermarket, buy your groceries, and all is good. Or you go out for dinner and order a meal, and all is good. The crazy thing that most people don't realise is that the foods we eat are all different. Where they come from is important, and the ingredients that are used in packaged foods or recipes or the way something is grown is much more important. For example, an apple from a supermarket might not actually contain the same nutrient density or goodness as an apple from a local farmer's market. So even though you are choosing to eat fruit—which most consider to be healthy—if it is grown using pesticides and chemicals, it's probably doing you more harm than good! Another example is an egg. An organic free-range egg contains a lot more omega-3 (good fats) and nutrient density than an egg from hens that are not cage-free and free-range.

We are the food our food ate. This means that not only are we what we eat, but the diet of the food we're eating will also affect us! When you eat eggs, you get the nutrients from the egg; and it's also important that the chicken that laid the egg was eating natural food options too, rather than artificial food and that the chicken's living environment is calm and clean. The same is true for all animal products. We should always aim for grass fed and organic where possible to get the best nutrition from our food. Grass-fed meat is much leaner than grain-fed meat, and the fat content it has is a much healthier form of fat. There are bundles of research about this kind of thing, and people like Dave Asprey, Gary Taubes, and Mark Sisson have done a lot of great work about educating the world on these topics. There are many more people who can guide us in this area. But the rabbit hole is deep; once you start digging, it will continue to unfold, and more information will come your way. Feel free to google these people and check out their masses of research.

This is extremely important. I could give you a meal plan or offer suggestions for how to create your daily intake, but if I don't also give guidance on *where* to get your food or the quality the food should be, I believe I'm doing you a disservice. It is up to you to what level you choose to pursue this journey, if at all. But I believe people should have all the information so they can make the best-educated decision in any situation, to set them up for long-term success and the ability to optimise their health. How far you take your research straightaway may depend on where you're at on your journey right now. For many, it might be a step-by-step journey to reaching optimal nutrition and health, and some may choose never to go there with regard to food quality.

For many, once we have knowledge, we know how powerful that knowledge is. We are hungry to keep learning in order to make the best decisions possible about food sources. My husband and I always avoid gluten and aim for dairy free wherever possible, as we can tolerate it in small amounts. We also try to minimise our intake of refined sugars (processed and packaged foods) as much as possible. We rarely drink alcohol and only occasionally drink caffeine. The reason we minimise what we have affectionately nicknamed the "fun five" is inflammation. We have found that we, and the thousands of people we've worked with over the years, benefit from reducing or swapping out these foods, both during their one-month detox phase and throughout life.

Inflammation negatively affects our gut health, our cells, our absorption of nutrients, our mood, our brain function, our hormones, and our emotions—and these might be just the short-term effects. If these issues continue long term and become chronic, they can lead to all sorts of nasty diseases later in life, like type 2 diabetes, heart disease, obesity, and maybe even cancer. We discuss these issues in more detail in many of our podcasts, so feel free to head to iTunes or stitcher to check out *The Chief Life podcast* and find out more (we have a podcast epsiode on gluten/dairy (episode 100), one on sugar (episode 104), and one on caffeine (episode 101). At the time of this writing, we have not recorded one for alcohol, but it is definitely on the horizon.

Prevention is the best medicine

The following are a few food groups to watch out for. It is important to know where these foods should be sourced from!

- *Fruit* – Organic, locally grown, and naturally in season is best. Most importantly, berries should be organic. It is less important for fruit with skin on it to be organic, as you can remove the skin; for example, with bananas, we don't consume the skin and, therefore, are protected from harmful pesticides that may be on the surface. With foods where you are likely to eat the skin (like apples and pears), it is better to buy organic or remove the skin, again to reduce intake of harmful pesticides and chemicals.
- *Vegetables* – Organic, locally grown, and naturally in season is best. Most importantly, leafy greens should be organic.
- *Fish* – Wild caught is best. Or if you have access to sustainably farmed fish, where the proprietors know exactly what is going into the feed and how the fish are looked after, this can also be an option.
- *Meat* – Grass-fed, free-range meat is best. Even better is organic meat. But if the latter is not possible, make grass-fed a priority.
- *Poultry and eggs* – Free range is best. If you can have your own chickens in your garden, even better! However, this won't work for everyone. Perhaps you might visit a local farmers market or research the eggs at your local grocery store.

This is a massive topic, and somewhat outside the scope of this book. However, much excellent research and many great books on these topics are available. The main takeaways from this section are:

- Buy grass-fed meat and eggs.

- Buy organic fresh produce if you can afford it or at least buy seasonal and local, and maybe ask whether the farmers use chemicals on the food grown.
- Wash your fruit and veg in iodine solution.
- Avoid foods that are processed, packaged, or high in inflammatory ingredients as much as possible (sugar, grains, dairy, alcohol, and caffeine; for some people, lectins, salicylates, amines, and other specific groups may need to be removed, but we recommend working with a healthcare professional for these more challenging groups).

Activity 4.1: Where Does Your Food Come From?

It's important to know not only where you are going to buy your food, but also where it has been prior to its arrival in the shop you buy it from. Questions to ask:

- Where does/do the meat/fish/chicken/eggs come from?
- How are the animals raised?
- Where are the fruit and vegetables sourced?
- Are herbicides and pesticides used?
- Who grew this food? What farm is it from?
- Is it certified organic? If not, how was it grown?
- What's in season at the moment?
- What do you mean by spray-free?

MODULE 2

Polishing

Review: Are You on Track?

It's time to check in with yourself. How did you do with sticking to your goals? Are they specific? Measurable? Achievable? Related to your long-term outcome? And have you set yourself a timeline to achieve them by? Giving yourself one or two weekly or monthly goals will help you to stay on track. It's also good to have a backup or emergency plan if things don't always go as anticipated (and it's extremely likely they won't always go as you think they will). You don't want to be left hungry with no food ready to eat, or you'll end up grabbing something that takes you further away from health and healing.

Carrying an emergency *snack attack pack* with you in your bag or car will assist with unprepared snack times. A great combination is a tin of tuna OR beef jerky, an apple, and a small handful of nuts. This covers all three macronutrients, requires no refrigeration, and will help curb any sugar cravings or 3:00 p.m. slumps to get you through to dinner when you get home.

Many of our clients over the years say, I've fallen off the wagon, and I need to get back on! I like to use a different analogy. Let's say there is no on or off the wagon. Instead, I prefer to say, ignore the wagon; stand on your own two feet; and, every time you need to make a health- or food-related decision, imagine you're standing at a fork in a road. As an adult, you get to choose whether you take the path that gets you closer to your goal, to health, and to thriving more in life with a fulfilling and pleasant outcome (because you are what you eat, and healthy wholesome nutritious foods will leave us feeling awesome). The other way is to choose to take yourself further away from your goals, further from health, and closer to disease—toward discomfort and a life of surviving, rather than thriving (because sugary processed foods and alcoholic or caffeinated beverages affect our hormones, gut health, and inflammation within the cells in our bodies, which affect our mood, digestion, nutrient absorption, and so much more). You have this choice every single time!

Hopefully, no one is holding you ransom and telling you that you have to eat or drink a certain thing. Peer pressure is real, and often we oblige others by eating and drinking certain things to feel accepted or to please them because they are asking you to or because they made it especially for you. At the end of the day, you know how you feel, and you are in charge of you. Intuitively, after living The Chief Life for a while, you will start to understand what foods and drinks do and don't agree with you, leading to better choices for your health and your higher self.

In the meantime, if that doesn't resonate, follow the principles. When you own your decisions, others are less likely to pressure you into a poor choice. On the other hand, if you go on about this diet you have to do because you're part of a challenge at your gym for only a short period of time, people will know you're not doing it because you want to do it and are more likely to harass you to break the rules. This then leaves you feeling like you've failed, and the downward spiral begins. Let's not go down that path hey! If you do choose to eat or drink something that is less favourable, remember that it is a conscious adult decision that you made. Own it, enjoy it, and then move on. Get back onto the path that takes you closer to your goals from your next meal, snack, or beverage. Make sense? *There is no wagon*, only you on your own two feet.

6

Balance Your Hormones

The type of foods we eat not only affect our external appearance but also have a huge impact on our hormones and chemicals internally. Eating the right foods provides us with more energy, aids sleep, improves skin, and increases muscle to fat ratio! Eat less favourable foods, and all the chemicals (additives, preservatives, allergens, inflammatory cytokines) turn our bodies into tired, overweight, and unproductive zombies that "wish" they could be more like the bouncy, energetic people who always seem so motivated. You can be that person! You just need to put in a little effort at the start, follow the principles, and watch the changes and awesome results happen.

However, you cannot out-train a bad diet, or as I prefer to say, less favourable nutrition choices (language and the way we phrase things is important because if we use the word "bad", we might start to think we are a "bad" person for eating a certain food, which lowers self-esteem and self-worth. By changing the way we talk to ourselves, we can change the way we feel about ourselves too – powerful stuff!). As much as you *want* to believe that you can go running for half an hour and burn off the calories from the pizza and beer you had the night before, it doesn't work like that. Calories *in* (consumed) do not precisely match up to equal calories *out* (expended). Over a lifetime of many years of nutritional abuse and eating unfavourable foods in excessive quantities, our insides will not be looking so happy, and we increase our risk of developing diseases and conditions such as type 2 diabetes or heart disease.

Prevention is *much* better than treatment, so my goal is to educate people/you to eat for health, well-being and quality of life, rather than thinking of food as a privilege. Food is a fuel and should be treated thus; eat the best quality foods in portion-controlled amounts to fuel your human body machine optimally. Yes, occasional treats are allowed and encouraged, but it's much harder to undo years of abuse than it is to practice avoidance and indulge occasionally.

Here's my suggestion for what has been extremely successful for myself and many of our thousands of past and current clients:

> Follow the rule of three macronutrients, every three to five hours in a balanced ratio (30 per cent protein, 40 per cent carbohydrates, and 30 per cent fats) as close to 90 to 100 per cent of the time as possible. (We aim for following these principles, most of the time, from Sunday morning through to Saturday dinner.)

> Then on a Saturday night, choose one (yup, that's right *one*) item—maybe a glass of wine *or* a dessert (for example, COYO

ice cream is a go-to for us because it still complies with our gluten and dairy-free food intolerance needs, with only a small amount of natural sugar being the vice).

We enjoy the treat with no guilt because we have *chosen* to eat it (conscious adult decision, not emotional eating or abuse of yourself). Then we wake up Sunday morning ready to get back on the healthful path because we may be a little swollen or inflamed from the treat the night before, leaving us feeling around a 5 to 7 out of 10, rather than our usual 9 to 10 out of 10. This makes us want to get straight back to eating balanced meals and snacks from healthy real food again.

Sometimes we get to Saturday night and don't even feel like having the treat, which is also fine. Knowing you have the choice can help to keep you sane and act as a mental health food or drink to allow you to still feel human and enjoy certain foods and drinks that you wouldn't normally have.

Our biggest advice, though, is to not be weird about it! Ha ha. If you do have a special occasion or a one-off social event where the food or drink may be out of your control, consider pre-ordering a gluten and/or dairy free substitute. Enjoy the event without making a big deal out of the fact that you might be eating differently from others. If it's normal for us and we just take it in our stride, others won't make a big deal either. People don't like *different*, they don't understand why you're not drinking alcohol because your ability to abstain and show willpower in the best interest of *your* health makes *them* feel bad—well, sorry, not sorry! Ha ha ha.

Your health is more important to you and me than their feelings—preventing cancer, heart disease, liver failure, and diabetes are much more important to you and me than their feelings. And we're not saying don't care what your loved ones think of what you're doing; if they love you, they should support your choices. If they don't understand it yet, sit them down and have a powerful conversation with them to explain what you are doing and why you are making these changes. It's best to do this at a quiet time that isn't at the actual social event to ensure you have their full attention.

So, in short, if you want to indulge—*do it*. Don't feel guilty, but still aim to follow your intolerance guidelines to look after your body. What I mean by this is that if you know you are intolerant to gluten or dairy, it is still recommended that you stay away from those foods 100% of the time, but if you choose to indulge, go for a gluten and dairy free option. If you want to stay on track—*do it*. But don't feel you have to explain yourself to anyone. Just plan ahead without making an issue about it to anyone else.

Activity 6.1: Emergency Action Plan

(Example of going out and how to plan ahead for it)

Temptation and date	What would I normally do?	Action plan to improve
Example Wedding on July 21	- Drink until I vomit - Eat whatever I want (the see-food and eat it diet, ha ha)	- Limit to five drinks (vodka lime and soda) with water between each - Have all three macros - Stay gluten and dairy free

Reassess this regularly, based on upcoming events and commitments, to best set yourself up for success. Make this a monthly or bimonthly activity by setting a reminder in your calendar.

7

Be Accountable: The Buddy System

Surrounding yourself with those who will support you through a lifestyle change is one of the key actions for success. Positive energy will allow you a much higher chance to achieve your goals and find more joy through this journey.

You are the average of the five people you surround yourself with. It's important to make sure you're spending time with people who lift you up rather than bring you down, who love you no matter what, who care about your health and well-being, and who are people that you want to be more like.

If you are surrounded by negative people, with negative energy, always naysaying and sapping the life out of you and everyone around you, remove them from your immediate world. You will notice straightaway how much better you feel and how much easier it is to focus on the things that make you feel good and the things that help you get closer to your goals!

The buddy system encourages you to find at least one other person, who may or may not want to be on this lifestyle change journey with you, to be there for you when you make a small (or big) win that you want to share so it is positively reinforced. This person can be a support to you when you feel weak and are considering straying from the path that takes you closer to your goals (no wagon remember, ha ha) before the event, not as confessions after! Use your buddy to help stop you from straying, not to own up to straying once you've already done it and are beating yourself up about it unnecessarily. This friend can remind you how amazing you are and that you are choosing to take part in this change to be a better version of *you*!

We usually suggest that your buddy is not your spouse, boyfriend, girlfriend, mother, father, sibling, best friend, offspring, or any other family member. This is because discussions can sometimes end in fights when your loved ones start behaving like a police officer around the house and making you feel guilty when you actually have made a conscious decision to stray and are okay with that decision.

If you can't find anyone or would rather meet some new people to assist you on this journey, feel free to join our core members' exclusive Facebook page. Please reach out to us to find out how to join (www.thechieflife.com/contact).

The best thing to do is find an inspiring and supportive friend who may have more of an interest in health and fitness. This friend will encourage you, rather than derail you (as sometimes your loved ones may inadvertently even enable you). For example, if you feel like ice cream and you tell your buddy, he or she should ask you a series of questions, like:

- *Why do you want some ice cream?* Think about it. Are you even actually hungry? Or are you just bored? Or is it coming up to that time of the month (ladies), and you think you're just craving sugar and comfort from the reward response?

- *Do you really want it? Or do you want something else?* Are you looking for attention or affection? Are you trying to avoid doing something or feeling something and looking for a quick-fix endorphin release type of distraction, which may actually leave you feeling more down afterward anyway?

- *What do you want most? What is your goal? What are you working towards? Is this taking you closer to your goal or further away?* You have a choice in every scenario—do you want pain (which, in this case, is the discomfort of choosing a less favourable food) or gain (which, in this case, is not choosing the less favourable food and getting closer to your goals)? If the food in question will actually take you further from your goal, it will cause you pain in the long term, so it's not really worth it, is it!? If you love and respect yourself, it's important to focus on what you want *most* (long-term goal), not what you want *now* (the ice cream).

Activity 7.1: Find a Buddy

Write down criteria for the kind of buddy you're looking for. Make a list of the names of people who would be good candidates. Number them in order from one upward, one being first choice. Then ask the first person on the list, using the following guidelines (this is a loose suggestion, and if you feel comfortable to have this conversation without any guidelines, go for it! This is just to assist those who might not have done something like this before):

> Hey, Bob,
>
> I'm about to embark on a health transition and would really appreciate it if you could be my support person for a few weeks whilst I get used to my new habits and way of eating. Would you be open to this? No worries if not, but I feel like you've been a great support to me and a super inspiring person in my life, so just thought I'd ask. All it involves is being available if I need to message or call you to help keep me on track. And maybe we can eat a few of the meals together; I'd be happy to cook them for us.

If the person says no, that's no problem. Ask the next person on the list! Consider asking someone from your gym or a colleague at work, these people might be more likely to have common interests and want to help you succeed.

MODULE 3

The Works

CHAPTER

8

Dial It Up and Dial It In: Portion Control

This is all about getting the right *quantity* of food, not only throughout the day but also at each meal. By eating the correct amount of food throughout the day and even thinking about the ratio of each of the macronutrient groups at each meal and snack, you can ensure you're getting the absolute most out of the way you fuel your body, as well as decreasing risk of diseases and negative health conditions farther down the track.

To work out how much energy you need for the whole day, use this basic energy equation:

Owen equation
Men: kcal/day = 879 + 10.2 × (weight in kg)
Women: kcal/day = 795 + 7.2 × (weight in kg)

Once you know how much you need for the whole day as your basic basal metabolic rate (BMR), we need to calculate how much of each macronutrient you need for the whole day and then at each meal and snack:

> *For fat loss*, take the calories for the day and add 300 to 500 calories depending on how much you train. For example, one hour of high-intensity exercise will require adding about 500 calories on top of the BMR calculated above.
>
> Remember, 30 per cent of your calories are to come from good quality protein, 40 per cent from good quality carbohydrates, and 30 per cent from good quality fats:
>
> Total calories × 0.3 for protein and fat
>
> Total calories × 0.4 for carbohydrates
>
> To calculate how many grams of each macronutrient you need for the day:
>
> Total calories × 0.3 / 4 g for protein = grams of protein needed for the whole day
>
> Total calories × 0.4 / 4 g for carbs = grams of carbohydrate needed for whole day
>
> Total calories × 0.3 / 9 g for fats = grams of carbohydrate for whole day
>
> It's best to create meals and snacks that are reasonably balanced in each of the three macros throughout the day.

For increased energy, add on about 600 to 800 extra calories and then repeat the calculations to figure out how many grams of each macro you need.

For muscle gain, add on about 900 to 1,100 extra calories and then repeat the calculations to figure out how many grams of each macro you need.

Use an app or website, like MyFitnessPal, to figure out the foods you can use to hit the numbers you have calculated. You can use some of the meals and snacks from the last module, enter them in, and see how much you might need to change the daily intake to hit your numbers more closely. You're aiming to be within 5 grams either side of each macronutrient per day to achieve absolute optimal results but this isn't essential; it's just for those who really want to take things up a notch!

Following this is the 7 Pillars of Health assessment sheet. This is an amazing way to see if all areas of your health are on track and how you might be able to adjust them to really optimise your health and results. Reset your goals in module 1 if you'd prefer to utilise this assessment as your weekly check-in instead of the numbers on the scales or body fat percentages, as sometimes we get so fixated on the numbers, we lose sight of what is actually important. We care more about how you feel and what you can do, rather than what you look like. And when the focus shifts, you naturally lean up and get a healthier body composition as a by-product.

Activity 8.1: All pieces of the Puzzle: Lifestyle Assessment

The Chief Life: 7 Pillars of Health Assessment

(Please circle the number that applies to you for each question below.)

1. **Nutrition/food/nourishment (including limiting alcohol)**

   I'm 100% = 0   75% = 1   50% = 2   25% = 3   Not on at all = 4

2. **Training/exercise/activity**

   Move daily = 0   5–6 days = 1   3–4 days = 2   1–2 days = 3   No movement = 4

3. **SLEEP**

   9 hours+ = 0   7.5 hours = 1   6 hours = 2   4.5 hours = 3   3 or less = 4

4. **Stress management/mindset**

   A. Deal with stress well = 0   Sometimes stressed = 2   Always stressed or anxious = 4

   B. Mostly positive = 0   Up and down = 2   Always down or find things hard = 4

5. **Hydration:**

   A. 3+ L/day = 0   2–3 L/day = 1   1–2 L/day = 2   .5–1 L/day = 3   <500 ml = 4

   B. No caffeine = 0   1/day = 1   2/day = 2   3/day = 3   4+/day = 4

6. **Vitamin D / sunshine / outside time**

   At least 30 mins outside/day = 0   10–20 mins/day = 2   No outside time/day = 4

7. **Breathing**

   A. Constant awareness of breath = 0   Daily breath exercises = 2   No awareness of breath = 4

B. Daily meditation = 0   Weekly meditation = 2   No meditation = 4

My score is: _____

Score Analysis

15 = on track   Score of 16–29 = changes   Score of 30+ = changes
                              may be needed   highly recommended

Main areas of focus for improvement:

Action plan for change:

How did you do?

The lower the score the better. For more details on how to assess your 7 Pillars of Health please watch the FAQ video about The Chief Life 7 Pillars of Health at https://youtu.be/Xti1ihcHifk.

A score below 15 means you're looking good and don't need to make too many adjustments!

A score between 15 and 30 means you should take a closer look at your current habits and possibly make a few amendments to help you reach a healthier and happier version of yourself.

A score above 30 means you're in trouble and definitely need to take a break or give yourself a chance to assess what's really important so you can focus on your number one asset—your *health*—and get this back on track so you can give more to the other areas of your life, like our family, work, hobbies, friends, and so on.

9

The Right Focus: Mindset

Keeping your head in the game is a massive part of the whole process. "The Right Focus" includes a few things to consider when it comes to mindset and shifting focus to ensure you are allowing yourself to succeed, rather than self-sabotaging.

Dos and don'ts

The concept is not thinking about what you can't have, as you only think about the subject and feel deprived. Rather than focusing on what you can't have, think about going from meal to meal. This will be easier to digest in bite-sized, step-by-step pieces, rather than a full, overwhelming four-week challenge. Think about what you want most, rather than what you want now. Also, remind yourself that this is your choice. You are choosing to do this; remember this instead of feeling deprived, limited, and powerless. Rather than saying, I can't, which is extremely limiting, maybe try saying, I'm choosing not to. The latter is a more empowering and owned belief system. You can also use the language of "swapping", as in "I will swap coffee for herbal tea" – this helps you to feel like you still have options when making changes to your current routine.

Integrity

Every time you start a challenge and give in or give up, it may be a lack of self-integrity. Try to align yourself with your goals and the things you want to achieve in your life. In the gym, integrity is completing all your reps or moving with good technique. In this case, we refer to integrity as doing the right thing even when no one is watching, for you and your optimal health.

Accept where you are

You are where you are because of what you've done so far and the choices you've made to date. You have a heartbeat, control of your hands, and control of what goes into your mouth. After reading this book, you will have the knowledge and understanding of *how* to put it all into practice. Moving forward, you can make the choices to get where you want to be.

Priorities versus excuses

We're all super busy these days and connected to everything at all times—thanks to our phones, computers, iPads, and other devices. But are you *busy*? Or do you not prioritise your health enough? It's easy enough to say you don't have time for something when you don't really want it; this is what we call an excuse. When you really want something to happen, you will make it a priority and take the necessary steps to improve and achieve your goals. Failing to plan is planning to fail! Food prep will set you up for success. Always being one step ahead and knowing where your next meal or snack is coming from will prevent you from making poor food choices. This may come across as confrontational, but it's important to be honest with yourself and give yourself permission to succeed. You deserve it!

Immune disorders and sickness

You may have a diagnosed illness, disease, or health issue. However, this shouldn't be your reason to prevent yourself from doing what you have control over to improve and achieve an improved health outcome. Food is fuel and medicine; it's about finding what fuel works for you and helps to prevent further development of negative symptoms. For example, you may have an underactive thyroid – like me, but this does not need to be the reason for you being overweight; if you are consuming ten cans of soft drink a day and eating fast food for every meal, this will lead to fat gain and health issues. If you choose to eat using the principles in this book, you will optimise your health and well-being, as well as your quality of life and possibly even reduce your autoimmune symptoms. Please seek out and work with a healthcare professional if you have been diagnosed with any specific issues.

Self-sabotage

Rewarding yourself for a good day with bad food is not actually a reward. It's self-sabotage. We all have that voice of self-doubt in our minds that leads us to believe the results we desire are unattainable. So we cheat on our diets and end up moving further from the goal because we believe we don't deserve it or will never reach it. Be kind to yourself and give yourself permission to succeed. Be your own biggest cheerleader and reward good behaviour with more good behaviour. This also links back to our belief systems from an earlier section in the book. You might take some time to write down your triggers and maybe what foods you tend to go for when you're emotionally charged, rather than for fuel or pleasure. Then you might limit these foods in the house (out of sight, out of mind or, in other words, remove the temptation). You might use your buddy system and/or come back to the questions you can ask yourself to prevent you from eating the foods that take you further from your goals. You might even have some new habits in place to use when you do get cravings or start to feel challenged by less favourable choices, like going for a walk, watching a comedy, listening to music that makes you happy and dancing around the house or calling a supportive friend.

Language

How we talk to ourselves and even the words we use to describe certain things in our lives can really mould the way we think about situations and define outcomes. For example, if we say, I'm such a bad person for eating or drinking "X", I'm awful – we end up feeling worse. This is because our words reinforce a negative view of ourselves, as well as releasing all sorts of negative hormones into our bodies, like cortisol and adrenaline. Another example is saying that foods are *good* or *bad*. We like to use *favourable* and *unfavourable* or *less favourable* instead.

If you beat yourself up with the words you use, it only reinforces the bad. It's a *fixed* mindset approach and something we should strive to change when we catch ourselves. Having a growth mindset in the way we speak to others and ourselves and the words we choose to use means we set ourselves up for success and allow more positive outcomes and reinforcements. You can learn more about fixed versus growth mindsets in the book *Mindset* by Carol Dweck.

Activity 9.1: Attitude of Gratitude

Try keeping a journal—starting tomorrow—when you first wake up as part of your morning routine. Write your schedule for the day, including when you plan to eat and roughly what you plan to eat (like a pre-emptive food diary). Then before bed, reflect as you tick off everything you've achieved for the day, especially if you followed the eating plan, using the schedule you had planned out for the day.

Follow these steps:

1. Buy a nice journal.
2. Buy a nice pen.
3. Place journal and pen somewhere next to your bed or where you will see it as soon as you wake up each morning.
4. Set your morning alarm to say, "Write in journal," or have a sticky note somewhere you will see when you first wake to remind you to write.
5. Open to a new page, write today's date and "I am thankful for" at the top of the page or whatever words come to mind that feel natural for you. Below this write one to three things you are thankful or grateful for. It can be anything, big or small, important or seemingly silly; just focus on things

that bring you joy and make you appreciate what you have going for you in this moment right now.

6. Below this write "Schedule." Jot down your rough schedule for the day, including when your meals and snacks will fit in, maybe even writing "what" you will be eating at each of those meals and snacks to ensure you're ready for the day ahead.

7. Go enjoy your day.

8. Set an alarm to remind you to start your bedtime routine—screens off, switch on gentle music, light a candle, have a shower, have a chamomile or other herbal tea, brush teeth, turn off bright lights, read a book, meditate (just choose the options that feel right for you; a bedtime wind-down routine can be anywhere from five minutes to thirty minutes to help you get ready for a good night's sleep). Finally—most importantly—when sitting in bed, open up your journal and reflect on wins for the day and something you might be able to improve on tomorrow. Feel free to tick off all the sections of your schedule you successfully achieved.

9. Sleep well, allowing yourself six, seven and a half, or nine hours of sleep to help you wake up feeling refreshed, well rested, and energised (as sleep cycles are about 90 minutes long, more about this in The Chief Life podcast episode 40 with the sleep doctor).

MODULE 4

New Habits

Success from Balance: The 80/20 Rule

Making this work long term means having a life whilst still following the main concepts of *Living The Chief Life*.

Activity 10.1 What Does Your Pie Chart Look Like?

Draw below how your 80/20 may look. We have provided an example for you to see, but your chart will be personal to you and so may look very different!

Example

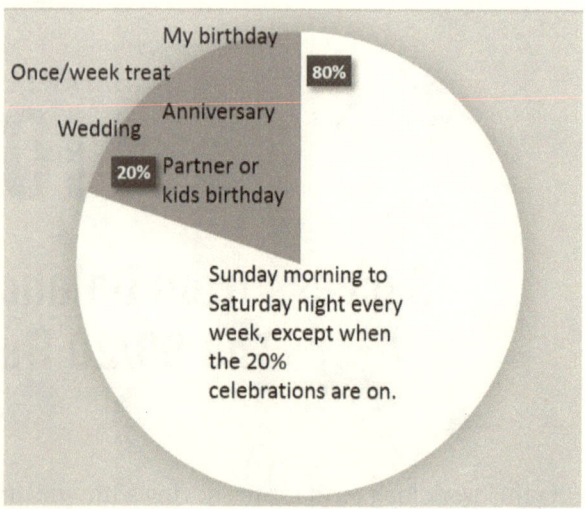

Your Pie Chart:

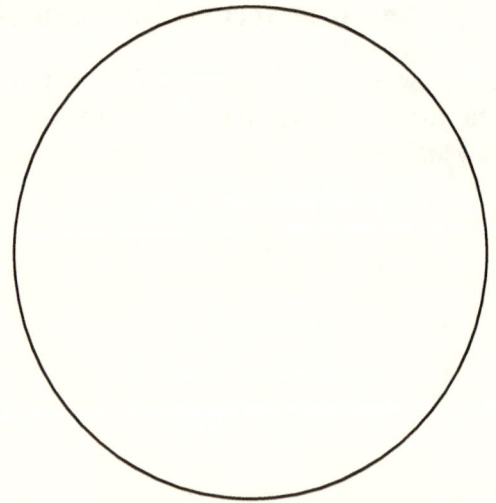

Long-Term Change Using Checkpoints

Activity 11.1: Refocus Your Goals / Realign Your Why!

Now that you're seeing some change, it's important to check back in with yourself periodically to make sure your progress is still headed in the right direction and that your current plan supports your current goals. As we have done throughout this process, setting dates to check back in with yourself is super beneficial and will continue to keep you on your path toward your destination, rather than drifting further away. As cliché as it is, it's about the journey, not the destination. If we put more focus on the now and each step of the way, finding joy in all the things we do each day, even if they seem mundane, we will get to the destination in a happy mindset. We won't be bothered about the end point. We will be able to get there with less discomfort and fewer issues. We might even arrive feeling like we got there faster. We will then be able to set a new goal to allow us to enjoy the next small chapter of the story of our lives.

So, what now? As you've almost reached the end of this book, I'd love for you to assess and reflect whether you've achieved what you set out to achieve and if you need to change direction or continue on the same path.

So far, I have intended to guide you with easy-to-follow steps to allow you to start making some changes. Moving forward, you'll need to find ways to keep yourself moving in the direction you want to be and keeping yourself accountable. Friendship circles, coaches and mentors are great for this, but setting up self-accountability systems is very valuable too!

Check out the flow chart that follows. It's an example of how a flow chart can help you assess whether you've achieved your current short-term body composition goals and what direction to take next as you set some new goals around body composition. If this wasn't the focus for you, use different words and create your own flow chart. For example, using the 7 Pillars scorecard can be so useful as a short-term goal-setting tool to see what areas need more attention, focus, and energy and whether the number has decreased since the last time you checked in. Or maybe, if you're using gym performance as a marker, ask yourself if you have become stronger (use your lifts to measure this) or fitter (see whether your workout times have gotten faster).

This is a very basic flow chart, but it gives you an idea of two of the most common goals. The ideology behind this type of flow chart is to question yourself more deeply about where you are, what you want to achieve, and what you might need to change to continue to move closer to that vision. So even if neither fat loss or muscle gain are of interest to you, you might want to increase energy levels or increase focus/performance at work or in training. You can use a similar process of questioning to see what you might need to tweak or adjust to continue to get closer to your long-term goals. The ideology here is just to dig as deep as possible, and using a visual diagram can be *so* helpful for that!

The Flow Chart

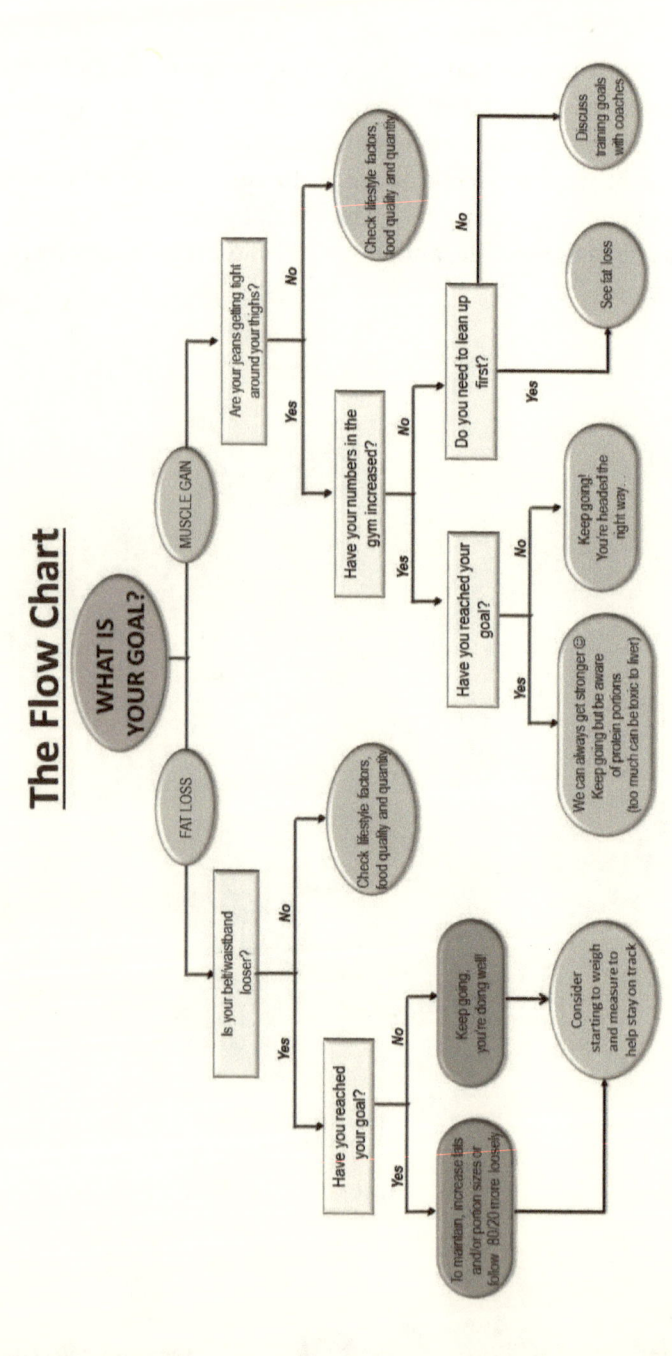

WHAT IS YOUR GOAL?

- FAT LOSS
- MUSCLE GAIN

FAT LOSS

Is your belt/waistband looser?

- **No** → Check lifestyle factors, food quality and quantity.
- **Yes** → Have you reached your goal?
  - **No** → Keep going, you're doing well! → Consider starting to weigh and measure to help stay on track
  - **Yes** → To maintain, increase bits and/or portion sizes or follow 80/20 more loosely. → Consider starting to weigh and measure to help stay on track

MUSCLE GAIN

Are your jeans getting tight around your thighs?

- **No** → Check lifestyle factors, food quality and quantity.
- **Yes** → Have your numbers in the gym increased?
  - **Yes** → Have you reached your goal?
    - **Yes** → We can always get stronger ☺ Keep going but be aware of protein portions (too much can be toxic to liver)
    - **No** → Keep going! You're headed the right way.
  - **No** → Do you need to lean up first?
    - **Yes** → See fat loss
    - **No** → Discuss training goals with coaches

Where to Next? Self-Guided Progress

Activity 12.1: Dream Storming and Journaling

The flow chart explored at the end of the previous chapter might not be your thing. So here is another example of a tool I like to use to explore where I'm at, reflect, and figure out what might need to be changed or let go of. Dream storming or journaling enables me to then set action plans to move forward using my imagination. This can be done by taking pen to paper or maybe even typing on a computer! You might prefer to draw or to chat about it with friends or loved ones before taking it to the written form. Whichever medium you choose, it might feel strange at first. But with time and practice, you'll find it's a fantastic way to dig deeper into your true self and pursue greater joy, meaning and happiness in life.

This exploration may be related to nutrition and health. Or perhaps it's more focused on life purpose and passion. I feel that all areas of our lives are linked, and we cannot be happy in one area if we are unhappy with another. For example, if we are unhappy in a relationship or job, we are much more likely to self-medicate with alcohol or emotionally abuse ourselves with unfavourable food choices.

How can we continue to make positive progress in our lives? By believing that we have a purpose, a vision, and a path to get there. Even if this path changes direction a few times or takes a few detours, that's okay (it's part of the journey). As long as we still feel like we're making headway, we can continue to feel like we matter.

There is an awesome book called *Tribe* by Sebastian Junger, which talks about homecoming and belonging. If you'd like to find out more about some of the following topics around community, it is a great place to start.

Something that has stayed with me and close to my heart for a while now are three areas that allow us to feel more worthy and of higher value to those around us and to ourselves— contribution, community, and connection:

> *Contribute* – If we feel we have something to bring to the rest of the world, we feel a sense of purpose and an ability to share with others.

> *Community* – To be part of something bigger than just ourselves is super important and reminds us we do not have to do this journey alone.

> *Connect* – Whether it be verbally, physically, emotionally, or spiritually, it is a wonderfully powerful thing to create a

deeper sense of self, not only with yourself but also with those you choose to surround yourself with.

Hopefully this gives you a starting point from which to build your foundations—a way to establish and build on your purpose and passion in life. We all want to feel like we have something to bring to this world and maybe even to leave behind, like a legacy. But it takes courage and choices to make sh*t happen and take action.

Spend some time free writing. This is literally just taking pen to paper and seeing what happens. Write whatever comes to mind, even if it seems odd, and just go with the flow. I find this especially useful after meditation or a yoga class, when I am fully present in my body and living from my heart and my intuition, allowing myself to express freely what I might need to pursue moving forward. Work with an energy healer or mentor or find a like-minded friend or family member to chat with so you can each explore your gifts and see how you might better contribute and connect with your community in order to build a greater awareness of what you can bring to the world in this lifetime.

Aim to make this a regular practice or ritual, although it should not feel like a chore. See if you can find a way to incorporate it into your life without it becoming a burden. I aim to do this daily, but sometimes it ends up being more like once a week, and that's okay too. Sometimes other things need attention, and creative writing or exploring your purpose might have to take a back seat. As long as you can make it a priority at least once a week or month, you'll receive the benefits of staying true to yourself and staying on your path of self-care and self-love.

A note on intuitive eating

I love educating people about food, health, and improving quality of life. Some of these things may be fact and based on science, and all of the information in this book is super powerful as a starting point to learn the basic principles of eating for health and well-being. Following this method will help to balance your hormones and allow you to tune in with your hunger and fullness signals (from ghrelin, the hunger hormone, and leptin, the satiation or satisfaction hormone). Certain foods will respond differently in different people and your body will give you signs and symptoms as to the foods that respond well and the ones that don't.

This is why it is very important to pay attention to how you feel when you eat and drink, as well as to how you respond in terms of mood, energy, feelings, and thoughts. The gut sends messages to the brain and vice versa. This is a skill that was innate and inbuilt in our ancestors. However, in modern ages, we have definitely disconnected from this more intuitive and connected way of listening to our bodies and our digestion.

I can give you all the science in the world, but what I really want to do is give you the tools and share enough of the basic knowledge with you so that you have the information you need to make better decisions about what you choose to put into your body moving forward.

This is not free reign to give yourself permission to eat anything and everything in sight just because you're choosing to. It's more about paying attention to what your body is asking you for. Eat when you're hungry, stop when you're full, know what keeps your energy and mood more evenly balanced, and eat in a way that brings you joy whilst also fuelling you in the best way possible to allow you to live a full and happy life.

Once you have followed the general suggestions from the meal plan / principles for about four to six weeks, you will start to get a sense of what works well for you and what doesn't work so well; you will have a grasp on how you can start to make food and drink choices based on feedback your body gives to you. Really check in with yourself. Be more present and more aware/mindful when you eat. Slowing down to eat your food will also help you to absorb more nutrients from your food, as well as keep you more calm, serving both your physical and mental health.

This can take time to develop, so you might start keeping a diary of how you feel after eating certain foods and drinking certain drinks and see what your body tells you. At the same time, though, try to stay relaxed and not overthink it all, as sometimes we can play tricks on ourselves. Use your gut instinct to guide you, rather than relying on your head to give you the answers.

Consider what brings you better health and internal long-term happiness versus what you are choosing to put into your body for short-term instant gratification or to please others' external expectations. Look after yourself inside and out and be confident in the decisions you make for yourself around nutrition and health.

Empower yourself.

When you do this, you will thrive. And you'll also inspire others to take a more nourishing and nurturing approach to food and their own health.

Success Stories

JW – Work-life balance

JW came to me for assistance with his nutrition to help him lose excess fat mass. Moreover, he had a goal of improving his long-term health and well-being. We started with a meal plan to help him learn the basics around meal timing and quality and quantity of food and then looked at his lifestyle more broadly to help him pinpoint some areas of stress that were impacting his progress.

Working a busy and stressful job that impeded on his training time, his downtime, and his family time was having a massive impact on his overall quality of life and his health outcome. For many people, it's not realistic to say, Just quit your job! Remove the stressful job and you'll be fine! People still need to earn a living, so running away from the problem is not always the solution.

JW and I worked together to help develop strategies and use various mindset tools to help him learn how to manage his stress and find more balance in his everyday life. We talked about bringing in rituals and frequent short breaks to help him feel less overwhelmed and set up boundaries (or freedom fences) to help him feel safe when bombarded with negative or stressful situations around him.

We cannot predict what is going to happen to us each day, but we can choose how we respond and react to any given situation. Once JW started to work on finding his work-life balance, his cortisol levels started to reduce, and he was able to start shifting his stubborn fat layer around his midsection, as well as find more happiness in every day. He now spends more time doing things that bring him joy and spends more quality time with his family.

He shares regular updates with me, and we continue to work together to help maintain this balance. He says it's an ongoing journey. But he is happy to keep learning and developing all areas of the 7 Pillars of Health in order to keep feeling his best.

HB – Sugar addiction

When HB first came to me, she was addicted to sugar and finding it hard to ignore the daily cravings for sugar and lollies. She had tried so many crash diets and often starved herself by neglecting to eat, which ended up leading to regular binges. She shared with me that she didn't eat very much but did enjoy a few drinks each night, and her sweet tooth was driving her crazy.

Her energy levels were up and down all over the place. She felt like she needed a long nap most days when she got home from work. So because she felt energy-less, she would try to use caffeine and sugar to help pick her up again to be able to go to the gym or to have energy.

I put her onto an initial detox to swap out the fun five foods for four to six weeks. Within just a couple of weeks, her energy levels stabilised. She had more to give at work and in training. She was no longer craving sugar and didn't feel the need to use caffeine to lift her energy. Her mood had also improved, and as an added bonus, her waist circumference had started to decrease, helping her to feel more comfortable in her clothes and her skin.

After some time following her meal plan alone, HB decided to take advantage of the nutrition coaching service we offer at The Chief Life. This is an accountability program that allows the member to email with or chat with their own personal nutrition coach once a week. In this check-in, the coach can assist the client in tweaking his or her meal plan, as well as with any queries specific to the week ahead.

HB loves her weekly check-ins and gets a lot out of knowing she has someone in her corner who can support her and keep her on track long term. Not only do clients get the support, they also receive education so that they learn how to utilise our philosophy and principles on their own when they choose to stop working with their coach. HB also loves our seasonal menus and has a collection of our meal plans that she uses to allow for more variety from week to week whilst staying within the guidelines. She has such a good understanding of how to build the "puzzle" that she now creates her own recipes using a mixture of those she has ordered from us over the years.

WD – Fasting

WD reached out to us initially for a performance-based, muscle gain meal plan. He is lean and healthy, and his goals were more around wanting to increase his capacity in the gym. He is super proactive and will follow the plan, whilst also using his own initiative when needed to make the best choice in a situation where maybe there are less favourable options available.

After being on the improved energy meal plan focus to begin with and reaping the benefits of many personal bests in the gym, he reached out to us to ask about fasting. Intermittent fasting (IF) is a popular topic of interest these days, but it is not for everyone. WD is a member of our core private Facebook group and so he has the ability to ask us questions whenever he likes, 24/7. He mentioned that he had heard about IF and was trying it out, but he was feeling very low in energy and not getting through his workouts like he was when he was eating something before training.

My response to him was very personalised, as every one of us is different, and we have different needs. There is no one size fits all. Just like with our meal plans, meal timing needs to be looked at case by case. There are guidelines that can be used, but each individual will need to use his or her routine and preferences to figure this out. We often refer to the chronotypes that Dr Michael Breus introduced us to in the sleep podcasts we recorded with him (episode 40 and 75 of The Chief Life podcast), and so I asked WD which chronotype he is (the quiz to find out which one you are can be found at thepowerofwhenquiz.com). He told me he is a lion, and why he was struggling with fasting every morning instantly made sense to me.

Lions tend to need to eat first thing in the morning in order to thrive. They are hunters, and so they generally wake up hungry and ready to go. Once I shared this with him, and he started to have a snack before going to the gym each morning, he felt better and started to see improvements in the gym again. He said he hadn't realised just how much the chronotypes affect us. But now he knows; it makes so much sense to him, and he will be more cautious when implementing new protocols around meal timing and food changes.

My motto is often, "If it isn't broken, don't fix it". We know WD is better off eating before training. He is lean and healthy. And he has tried not eating before training and knows now that doesn't work for him. So he will stick with eating in the morning and not use the IF protocol. If he did want to shorten his eating window, he could just have dinner earlier. People often use this method to reduce their daily eating window down to eight to ten hours in order to let the gut rest for the rest of the day/night. I have seen benefits for both using this method and not using it, so again it will come down to personal preference and trial and error.

Matty, my husband, is a bear chronotype and does very well with fasting until about 10:00 or 11:00 a.m., whereas I am also a lion and, like WD, wake up hungry and ready to eat breakfast. WD is doing extremely well and is even doing some extra weightlifting technique training on top of his current exercise program, privately coached by Matty.

AF – Migraines

AF came to me originally regarding possible food intolerances that were causing excruciating migraines. We sat down for a face-to-face consult to dig deeper into what might be the problem. She was also keen to lean up a little, but that was not the main focus. Her migraines had started to become quite debilitating and were affecting both her personal life and her professional life.

She already ate reasonably healthfully and clean, with a few dairy and gluten foods sneaking in here and there and the occasional alcoholic drink. She was a healthy weight and trained regularly. I started her on the detox but a little stricter than normal—with wild-caught fish and grass-fed meat only to make sure we were really limiting inflammation from the foods she was eating. She became stricter with swapping out gluten and dairy, as these are extremely inflammatory to the four defence systems within the body (gut, brain, skin, and blood), as well as abstaining from alcohol and caffeine in order to see how she felt with removal of the fun five. Sugar was already pretty minimal, so she didn't find it hard to remove that completely.

She definitely felt a massive improvement by allowing her body a chance to heal naturally using this anti-inflammatory way of eating. We also spent a lot of time focusing on the other six pillars of health too. AF made sure she was getting a minimum of seven and a half hours sleep a night. She took more time outside in the sun each day, drank plenty of water, walked to and from work, and took regular breaks to decrease stress levels. She meditated and practicing yoga to help with her mindset and breath focus and got daily exercise in somehow—whether it was at the gym, yoga, or just the walk to and from work.

Again, she was feeling better. She had trimmed up a little, and her energy levels had improved. But she was still suffering from migraines, so we hadn't quite found the culprit yet! Then one morning, it suddenly hit me. There was something I hadn't really paid much attention to when in sessions with clients—what types of electronics they use or have around them at all times. We constantly have our mobile phones by our sides, in our pockets or handbags, and these send out electromagnetic frequencies (EMF) that can affect our own EMF signals. In this case, it wasn't her mobile phone, but the exercise watch she was wearing 24/7 apart from when she showered once a day. She wore the device on her left wrist, and the migraines were on the left side of her head.

AF had been to many doctors and specialists who had been unable to pinpoint what was affecting her. Some had even suggested it was all in her head—no pun intended here, as this is a serious matter!

I messaged AF as soon as I had my epiphany, and she took the watch straight off. She has not worn it since and has had no migraines since. Some people are much more susceptible to EMF signals from electronics than others, and this is a very specific and extreme case. Nevertheless, it illustrates something important to be aware of. You can follow the meal plan and pay attention to all of your health pillars, but sometimes what's ailing you or getting in your way is something a little more left field. It may take some thinking outside of the box to really figure out what is going on.

AF is feeling a million times better and is so thankful to me for helping her to identify this issue. She has continued to take care to avoid EMF wherever possible and still follows the principles and The Chief Life philosophy we live by. She takes time to care for herself and prioritises focus on her 7 Pillars of Health, and she is thriving.

***

Thank you for investing time, energy, and money into reading this book. Please share it with anyone you feel may also benefit from it. My aim is to continue spreading my love of health, well-being, and improved quality of life to all who I meet. In that process, I will hopefully bring more light and happiness, even where there may still be darkness and sadness. Balance is key, but live from a place of love, and you will live a full life. All my love, Stacey Lee Turner

APPENDIX

Meal Plan Examples

Example. Small female; goal, fat loss

Meal	Day 1	Day 2	Day 3
Meal 1	3 eggs 1 cup cooked spinach 1 cup tomato 1 cup cooked mushrooms 50 g sweet potato 3 tbsp avocado	Smoothie: 1 serve protein powder 150 ml coconut water 1.5 cups berries 1 tsp almond butter or 9 nuts Handful of ice Blended	3 eggs 1 cup cooked spinach 1 cup tomato 1 cup cooked mushrooms 50 g sweet potato 3 tbsp avocado
Snack 1	30 g meat 1/2 pear 3 cashews	1 boiled egg 1/2 apple 3 almonds	30 g meat 1/2 pear 3 cashews
Meal 2	90 g chicken or other lean meat 1 cup baby spinach 1 capsicum 1 small cucumber 1 medium carrot 1 cup celery 15 olives	135 g fish, cooked anyhow 3–4 cups cooked veg (broccoli, cauliflower, carrot, capsicum, eggplant, zucchini) 3 tbsp avocado	90 g chicken or other lean meat 1 cup baby spinach 1 capsicum 1 small cucumber 1 medium carrot 1 cup celery 1 tbsp olive oil
Snack 2	45 g smoked salmon 1 kiwi 3 walnuts	30 g chicken breast 1 mandarin 3 pistachios	1/2 small tin tuna 1 kiwi 3 walnuts
Meal 3	Mexican: 135 g minced meat 50 g tomato paste 1 carrot grated 1 cup chopped capsicum Large lettuce leaves 3 tbsp avocado Paprika Mexican spices	Chicken: 90 g chicken breast 3 cups roasted vegetables drizzled with cinnamon, salt, pepper, and olive oil *or* steamed vegetables with olive oil drizzled on plate	Curry: 90 g–135 g your choice protein 1 medium carrot 1 cup broccoli 1 cup cauliflower 1 cup capsicum 3 tbsp coconut milk 1 tsp curry powder 1 tsp allspice

Day 4	Day 5	Day 6	Day 7
Smoothie: 1 serve protein powder 150ml coconut water 1.5 cups berries 1 tsp almond butter or 9 nuts Handful of ice Blended	3 eggs 1 cup cooked spinach 1 cup tomato 1 cup cooked mushrooms 50 g sweet potato 3 tbsp avocado	Smoothie: 1 serve protein powder 150ml coconut water 1.5 cups berries 1 tsp almond butter or 9 nuts Handful of ice Blended	3 eggs 1 cup cooked spinach 1 cup tomato 1 cup cooked mushrooms 50g sweet potato 3 tbsp avocado
1 boiled egg 1/2 apple 3 almonds	30 g meat 1/2 pear 3 cashews	1 boiled egg 1/2 apple 3 almonds	30 g meat 1/2 pear 3 cashews
135 g fish, cooked anyhow 3–4 cups cooked veg (broccoli, cauliflower, carrot, capsicum, eggplant, zucchini) 3 tbsp avocado	90 g chicken or other lean meat 1 cup baby spinach 1 capsicum 1 small cucumber 1 medium carrot 1 cup celery 15 olives	135 g fish, cooked anyhow 3–4 cups cooked veg (broccoli, cauliflower, carrot, capsicum, eggplant, zucchini) 3 tbsp avocado	90 g chicken or other lean meat 1 cup baby spinach 1 capsicum 1 small cucumber 1 medium carrot 1 cup celery 1 tbsp olive oil
30 g chicken breast 1 mandarin 3 pistachios	45 g smoked salmon 1 kiwi 3 walnuts	30 g chicken breast 1 mandarin 3 pistachios	1/2 small tin tuna 1 kiwi 3 walnuts
Grilled fish: 135 g fish Roasted vegetables: 1 cup cauliflower 1 cup broccoli 1 cup zucchini 1 cup eggplant 1 tsp mayonnaise	Steak: 90 g steak vegetables drizzled with cinnamon, salt, pepper and olive oil *or* steamed vegetables with olive oil drizzled on plate	Stir-fry: 90 g–135 g your choice protein 1 medium carrot 1 cup broccoli 1 cup cauliflower 1 cup capsicum 9 cashews Paprika Chilli powder for a spicy touch	Seafood marinara: 135g seafood mix 1 carrot 1 cup broccoli 1 cup cauliflower 1 cup zucchini 50g tomato paste 3 tbsp coconut milk

Example. Large male; goal, improved energy and performance

Meal	Monday	Tuesday	Wednesday
Meal 1	5 eggs 1 cup spinach 1 cup tomatoes 1 cup mushrooms 1 cup capsicum 100 g sweet potato 5 tbsp avocado	Smoothie: 1.5 serves protein powder 150 ml coconut water 1 banana 1 cup berries 1.5 tsp almond butter Blended	5 eggs 1 cup spinach 1 cup tomatoes 1 cup mushrooms 1 cup capsicum 100 g sweet potato 5 tbsp avocado
Snack 1	60 g meat 1 pear 6 cashews	2 boiled eggs 1 apple 6 almonds	60 g meat 1 pear 6 cashews
Meal 2	150 g slow-cooked meat 140 g pumpkin 2 cups baby spinach 1 capsicum 1 small cucumber 1 medium carrot 1 cup celery 12 spears asparagus 2 tbsp olive oil	225 g fish or seafood 60 g cooked rice 4 cups cooked veggies (broccoli, cauliflower, capsicum, carrot, zucchini, eggplant) 5 tbsp avocado	150 g chicken 100 g sweet potato 2 cups baby spinach 1 capsicum 1 small cucumber 1 medium carrot 1 cup celery 12 spears asparagus 1 tbsp olive oil 10 olives
Snack 2	1 small tin tuna 1 pear 6 walnuts	20g beef jerky 2 mandarins or kiwis 6 pistachios	1 small tin tuna 1 pear 6 walnuts
Meal 3	Italian meatballs: 225 g meatballs 2 carrots grated 1 cup tomato 1 cup capsicum 1 cup zucchini spirals 50 g cooked gluten-free spaghetti pasta 5 tsp dairy-free cheese Italian mixed herbs	Sausage and mash: 225 g sausage 100 g sweet potato mash 3–4 cups roasted vegetables drizzled with cinnamon, salt, pepper, and extra olive oil	Stuffed capsicum: 150g beef 60g cooked rice 1 1/2 grated carrots 1 cup broccoli 1 cup cauliflower 1 cup capsicum 5 tsp dairy-free cheese Paprika Salt & Pepper

Thursday	Friday	Saturday	Sunday
Smoothie: 1.5 serves protein powder 150 ml coconut water 1 banana 1 cup berries 1.5 tsp almond butter Blended	5 eggs 1 cup spinach 1 cup tomatoes 1 cup mushrooms 1 cup capsicum 100 g sweet potato 5 tbsp avocado	Smoothie: 1.5 serves protein powder 150 ml coconut water 1 banana 1 cup berries 1.5 tsp almond butter Blended	5 eggs 1 cup spinach 1 cup tomatoes 1 cup mushrooms 1 cup capsicum 100 g sweet potato 5 tbsp avocado
2 boiled eggs 1 apple 6 almonds	60 g meat 1 pear 6 cashews	2 boiled eggs 1 apple 6 almonds	60 g meat 1 pear 6 cashews
225 g fish or seafood 80 g cooked quinoa 4 cups cooked veggies (broccoli, cauliflower, capsicum, carrot, zucchini, eggplant) 5 tbsp avocado	150 g slow-cooked meat 140g pumpkin 2 cups baby spinach 1 capsicum 1 small cucumber 1 medium carrot 1 cup celery 12 spears asparagus 2 tbsp olive oil	225 g fish or seafood 60 g cooked rice 4 cups cooked veggies (broccoli, cauliflower, capsicum, carrot, zucchini, eggplant) 5 tbsp avocado	150 g chicken 100 g sweet potato 2 cups baby spinach 1 capsicum 1 small cucumber 1 medium carrot 1 cup celery 12 spears asparagus 1 tbsp olive oil 10 olives
20 g beef jerky 2 mandarins or kiwis 6 pistachios	1 small tin tuna 1 pear 6 walnuts	20 g beef jerky 2 mandarins or kiwis 6 pistachios	1 small tin tuna 1 pear 6 walnuts
Kebabs: 150 g lamb kebabs 75 g pineapple pieces 50 g chickpea mash 2–3 cups mixed steamed vegetables with olive oil drizzled on plate 1 tbsp homemade garlic sauce	Shepherd's fish pie: 225 g tinned tuna or fish pieces 1 1/2 cups zucchini 1 1/2 cups carrot 1/3 cup peas 100 g sweet potato mash to top 1–2 tbsp homemade mayonnaise Salt & Pepper	Burger: 225 g mince patty 1 1/2 grated carrots 1/2 cup beetroot 1 1/2 cups capsicum 5 tbsp avocado In the mince: 1 clove garlic 1/2 onion, chopped 1 small gluten-free bun	Seafood stir-fry: 225 g seafood mix 50 g cooked vermicelli noodles 1 1/2 cups carrot 1 1/2 cups broccoli 1 1/2 cups cauliflower 1 cup zucchini 1/2 onion 1 cup beansprouts 15 cashews